Lucy,

To you perfect Health,

Ken NS

Wanakee's Nutritional Approach to Vitiligo & Other Autoimmune Diseases

---

A Traditional Naturopath's Personal Journey

Toward Healing Naturally

Wanakee Hill, N.D.

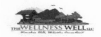

The Wellness Well Press

Mandeville, LA

USA

The Wellness Well Press

P O Box 862

Mandeville, LA 70471

www.thewellnesswell.net

www.wanakeehill.com

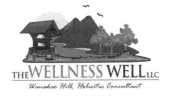

Note: This book is for nutritional and informational purposes only. It is not meant to diagnose, treat or prescribe. Please consult a medical doctor before using the information and supplements recommended in this book.

This book is dedicated to

My late mother, Mary, whose knowledge of natural remedies and quest for knowledge through books, gave me an early education and introduction to nutritional therapies that changed my life.

My husband, Michael D Hill, who said to me, "Follow your passion," which led to my Doctor of Naturopathy -- my lifelong dream.

A very special thank you to www.MichaelHillMedia.com for editing this book with tender loving care and journalistic expertise.

All the people I've encountered with vitiligo via VSIG, my vitiligo products and consulting company, or on the streets. You give me strength to continue on my path to healing. I learn as much from you as you learn from me.

Contents

———————

Chapter 1

Vitiligo

A traditional naturopath's personal story

I can never remember a time in my life when I didn't have vitiligo. From the age of 5 or so, I remember 2 white patches on my right thigh. I guess they were always there. In the summer, adults would often ask me if I was burned. My response always was, no, it grows when I grow.

In retrospect, the vitiligo was spreading as I grew. Small, erratic patches began cropping up around the original two. At about puberty, two vitiligo patches had become four, then six, with some uneven skin tones scattered about.

I recall repeatedly asking my mom to take me to the doctor. Her constant response was there's nothing they can do. What I didn't understand in her response was that she likely had tried to get help for my white patchy skin. There was none available to her.

I played carefree as a kid, yet mindful of my white spots. The older I got, the more self-conscious I became about my white patchy thigh. The stares, the pointing, and sometimes laughter, kept me from going to swimming classes in the summer. I remember keeping my arm and hand straight on my leg when I wore shorts -- my attempt at hiding the vitiligo and my personal shame. I honestly thought I was a leper!

At about age seventeen, I saw a team of doctors, thinking my mom didn't take this malady serious enough to find doctors to heal me. This team examined my vitiligo and told me its name. The doctors then told me that by the time I reached my 30s, this disease that was so emotionally crippling for me would be all over my body. I was devastated. I was offered nothing to treat the vitiligo. Worst of all, I was offered no hope of getting better. I was given only a dire prediction of getting worse -- much worse.

In high school, there was a tall female teacher who had uneven patches of skin. I always thought it must be vitiligo, though I never asked. I dreaded the thought of getting her age with noticeable uneven skin tone. There had to be something to help prevent this from happening to me. Those doctors had to be wrong.

I'm not the kind of person who gives up. So I left the team of doctors and went directly to the main library. I gathered huge medical text books. I remember seeing pictures of African children's bodies, riddled with vitiligo. Oh, the horror I felt. I studied as much as I could, and then vowed to fight vitiligo so that I would never look like the painful pictures I'd seen in those books. I knew it was time to go back to my roots.

My maternal grandmother was half Cherokee. My mom, like her mom before her, used natural remedies, passed down for generations. I grew up on medication only in emergencies. For every ailment, we used herbal and nutritionally based remedies. It was a way of life.

It goes without saying, my run-in with the medical profession took me home, literally and figuratively. My mom always mail-ordered healthful healing books. We had a steady supply arriving in my teen and young adult years. I read them all, absorbing the information like a sponge. I read one book that talked about a woman in California who made her own sun block, to protect her vitiligo from the sun, since she had been told the sun was harmful to vitiligo. She loved to sunbathe every day, so she mixed a B vitamin that is a natural sunscreen, with mayonnaise and put it on her vitiligo patches daily. What she didn't expect to happen was pigmentation – the return of color to her patches. She began to get freckles using the daily sunscreen.

This story really piqued my interest. I bought the tablets, crushed them as best I could, added them to olive oil and put the mixture on my skin. The next morning, my largest and oldest patch had a very noticeable freckle of color. I knew I was on the path to healing through nutrients and food.

For awhile, I followed through on the gritty mixture and gained even more freckles. My progress was slow, but steady. Eventually, summer turned into fall and I lost interest. Unless I was wearing shorts and getting stares or questions about being burned, I didn't pay much attention to my vitiligo for very long.

I wanted it gone, but the process of gaining a few freckles here and there with the homemade gritty mix was quite tedious. While I put this remedy aside temporarily, in the back of my mind, I knew I could do natural things to improve my condition.

A few years later, I married and noticed my hair was breaking, thinning and coarser. Also, I had cold hands and feet. It wasn't until I was in a bookstore with my father-in-law and thumbed though the glossary of a book did I realize I may have a thyroid problem. The symptoms certainly were there. I started researching thyroid issues and learned about Broda Barnes' basal temperature test. I had a temperature that was far less than 97.6, which my doctors never stated was a problem.

As a matter of fact, a nurse once seemed surprised that my temperature was up. The nurse asked if I was sick. She then said my current temperature was "normal for most," but unusually high for me! Still no focus on my thyroid, though the nurse suspected an infection-induced fever when my temperature appeared within near normal ranges in the late afternoon!

I did further research and decided to nourish my thyroid. Based on the symptoms, I doubted I was first-generation hypothyroid. Research shows generational thyroid conditions require more than iodine therapy.

My hair, skin and overall vitality seemed to respond immediately. I was so grateful for the book, the knowledge, and most of all, the relief.

I learned things from various sources that may be helpful to the thyroid, as well as some recommendations for vitiligo. I was well on my way to a natural healing regimen that I believe has helped to curb the spreading of vitiligo.

Once I started taking care of my thyroid, I noticed the vitiligo stopped spreading. What a relief. I seemed to have spreading at other times in my life, which included hormonal changes like puberty and at times of high stress.

After the death of my mother, I began to get a few vitiligo patches. I used the B vitamin solution to hopefully prevent full onset white in these patches. It seemed to have worked.

Now that I'm nearing the age of menopause, I have noticed a few patches recently. Stress and anxiety may have been contributors as well.

There are some similarities with vitiligo sufferers that research seems to back up. The thyroid is so often implicated in vitiligo sufferers that many practitioners now consider vitiligo a symptom of a malfunctioning thyroid.

For the many people who contact me about vitiligo, I always recommend getting the thyroid checked through blood tests and performing the Broda Barnes test. I honestly believe testing the thyroid is one of the most important recommendations for anyone who has vitiligo. Unless the endocrine system is functioning properly, it's virtually impossible to truly help to halt the spread of vitiligo, research shows.

The second most important issue that I emphasize in my vitiligo is diet. I always impress upon people the potential relationship among what we are eating, how we digest it and vitiligo.

Vitiligo sufferers tend to have low stomach acid. Further, nutrients such as B12, B6, folic acid, PABA, zinc, tyrosine, copper and vitamin C are often deficient in vitiligo sufferers. Vitiligo sufferers are shown to digest proteins poorly. Digestion is often less than adequate and so is nutrient absorption. The liver is implicated in vitiligo. Fats, carbohydrates and other undigested nutrients may encourage liver congestion. Supplements that relieve liver congestion are shown to help to reduce the size and number of vitiligo patches.

There are some indications that leaky gut syndrome may play a role in vitiligo. I am one who takes this theory seriously. There is a saying that all disease begins in the gut, meaning digestion plays a vital role in health, wellness and longevity.

Taking all of this information and using it to form the basis of a nutritionally oriented healing regimen for my vitiligo, I have witnessed the reduction in the size and numbers of my vitiligo patches. Staving off the spreading of the disease naturally is the method of choice for me, using nutrition, both internally and externally. Without the aggressive plan of action

I've chosen, I do believe my vitiligo would've spread, as predicted.

As a traditional naturopath who has followed this path all of my life, it was easy for me to gravitate toward a holistic healing approach to vitiligo. Research and evidence echoed the things I found to ring true in my own healing journey.

Through the years, research, trial and error, being a part of the Vitiligo Support and Information Group, or VSIG, I've learned a lot about my vitiligo and the vitiligo of others. I've come away with a strong belief that vitiligo is a disease that seems to respond most favorably to healthful living, whole foods, supplements, exercise and stress reduction.

This book is written for every person who struggles with vitiligo, their loved ones, caregivers, or anyone who wants to learn about taking control of his or her health through nutrition and balanced living, potentially bringing back skin color, as well as promoting a balanced and healthful body, mind and spirit.

I've talked to many people around the world who suffer with vitiligo. The recurring theme is one of depression, low self-esteem, frustration and a deep desire to rid their bodies of vitiligo.

My goal is to offer valuable, easy-to-follow information on what has worked for me as well as others who have journeyed the nutritional path to healing vitiligo.

I'm very disappointed to say more than 3 decades after I was told there's nothing you can do, parents and their young children, as well as older vitiligo sufferers are getting the exact same response today.

I'm here to proclaim, there is something you can do! You can empower yourself with knowledge on how to target imbalances within your body, which may promote healing. I'm here to promote health through proper eating, drinking and living.

A balanced, well-functioning body has the potential to correct and reverse ailments and heal itself. Ensuring your body, mind and spirit are nourished, balanced and well-tuned, seem key to ridding the body of diseases such as vitiligo.

This incurable disease that I once feared and that once conquered me is now one that is under control and healing, through the power of nature.

When I consult on vitiligo in my traditional naturopathic capacity, I offer a unique perspective: I'm a person who has struggled with the physical, emotional and psychological aspects of vitiligo --

which only a person who has the disease can fully understand.

When I say to my clients, I know what you're going through, I really mean it.

Chapter 2

The psychological effects of vitiligo:

Emotions, stress and self-loathing

There are many with vitiligo who are in full
acceptance of the disease. Many forget they have
vitiligo and are comfortable in their skin.

In my many conversations and consultations with
vitiligo sufferers, I have documented the recurring
theme of hating a specific part of their body
inflicted with vitiligo; hating their entire being or
just hating the fact that they have the disease. I have
noticed the added stress, strain and anguish that
people without this emotionally debilitating disease
can neither fully understand nor appreciate. The
burden of vitiligo acts as the self-imposed scarlet
letter for many of those who have it. It is an
outward sign of inward shame and disgust at the
disfigurement that seems so resistant to medication,
healing and wholeness.

In my practice, I spend a lot of time listening. My
clients are in pain. Vitiligo itself is not a physically
painful disease. There may be some itching when
the skin is actively losing color; however the
emotional pain of vitiligo is often so unbearable, its

sufferers retreat to a lonely life of hiding from the world. Socializing may be difficult. For some, leaving the house for anything other than work becomes a challenge. Relationships are sometimes impossible in extreme cases. Life, in general, is depressing and difficult for some people who are so repulsed by the disfigurement, that they project that sentiment onto the world at large. It doesn't help that people tend to stare or have misconceptions about vitiligo. That adds further emotional stress to a very stressful malady.

Stress is a potential danger to health in general, and is believed to exacerbate the effects of vitiligo in particular. Keeping stress low may help to reduce or prevent the spreading of vitiligo.

To lower stress, I try to eat healthfully, preferring whole and organic foods, with mineral-rich water, herbal teas and a generally high-alkaline diet, to ensure I'm getting the proper fuel for a healthful body, mind and spirit.

In addition to a healthful diet, I supplement to nourish my glands and use other healthful supplements to aid my body in dealing with stress. Reducing my overall stress level with exercise and incorporating homeopathy as a means of managing and reducing stress are an important part of my regimen.

Nutrition and supplements that may help to reduce stress may also help to balance emotions that are potentially detrimental to health, and potentially dangerous to those who suffer from vitiligo.

Anger, fear, depression, anxiety and other toxic emotions are shown to add stress and trauma to the immune system and body. Behavioral changes through modification, consultations, therapy sessions, meditation, deep breathing, hypnosis and other means, may prove helpful.

I have found homeopathic remedies to be quite beneficial to my regimen. In times of stress, homeopathy is a potentially wonderful tool; however, I believe the everyday stress that my mind, body and spirit undergo, inhibit the health of my vitiligo, as well as my overall health. I use homeopathy as a daily stress-relieving tonic, to prevent damage to my immune system and body, which may come from low-grade daily stress.

To heal, naturopathy teaches that we have to take a holistic approach, meaning we must look at body, mind and spirit.

Stress can have a major impact on our physical health, our mental outlook and mental health, as well as the health of our spirits. In addition to a daily homeopathic remedy to keep my daily stress to a minimum, so that my immune system will not have the extra burden of fighting off excess stress, I use a sublingual immune regulating protein supplement that is shown to balance immune response. Homeopathic pellets for the reduction of stress, which may benefit vitiligo as well as immune health in general, along with the thymus supplement, are available at www.TheWellnessWell.net.

Other supplements that may be helpful include a daily vitamin and mineral supplement.

Herbs may help to balance the immune system and potentially aid in correcting dysfunction that may contribute to vitiligo.

Stress may have a devastating effect on the adrenal glands, often leading to exhausted adrenals. Supplementing with raw glandulars may prove beneficial to vitiligo. These glandulars are available at www.TheWellnessWell.net.

Some of the ways I've handled stress is not allowing things to get to me, or shaking it off! This method has proven quite helpful, along with confronting stressful issues head on. I have begun to confront people who say or do things that are offensive or toxic to my well-being. As uncomfortable as it may be, it's better to get it out in the open and deal with it, rather than holding it in and suffering, causing further damage and stress to the body. If talking does not solve the problem, it is often a good idea to simply remove toxic people from your life. Explain to them why you feel it's best that all or most contact cease, if this is the only way to make peace with that person and your overall mental, physical and spiritual health.

Meditation, deep breathing, mentally going to your favorite relaxation spot or just focusing your mind on peace, tranquility and healing, are shown to help to alleviate stress and facilitate healing.

The least amount of tension and stress you hold inside, the less likely the stress may damage your health.

Do you clench your fists? Are your teeth often clenched? Do you have a high stress, type A personality? These are very dangerous signs of high stress and are a warning sign to take positive steps to reduce the stress in your life to improve your health.

Learning to deal with anger, resentment, envy, hostility or other negative emotions, situations and people takes time and may require professional help. In the long run, a happier, healthier, well adjusted life may be your reward!

How do you spell relief?

Kee's Health Tips ©

Stress is shown to have a major effect on illness, disease and ultimately, may contribute to premature death. Finding constructive ways of coping with stress is one of the most important things that I recommend for your health.

☐ **Emotions** – Anger, resentment, fear, hatred, unresolved tensions and holding things in, are quite detrimental to health. They are shown to pose many dangers. These emotions may burn, freeze or damage cells and store in organs, later manifesting as autoimmune diseases such as rheumatism, which is closely linked to vitiligo. Deal with these emotions. Don't hold them in. Take deep breaths. Count to 10. Walk away. Take a cold shower. Dance. Laugh.

Cry. Go into a private area and throw a temper tantrum.

☐ **People Power** – Surround yourself with positive people who bring out the best in you. Detoxify your life. Negative or toxic people are dangerous to your health and well-being. Happiness is contagious! Smile! Think happy thoughts.

☐ **Mimic Children** – Children are generally happy, carefree and full of energy. When emotions overwhelm them, they simply cry or throw a tantrum. While most adults may consider the behavior unacceptable, research shows children's methods of dealing with stress are quite healthful. Tears are filled with healing hormones, research shows.

☐ **Talk It Out** - Talk to yourself, a friend, a therapist, the wall or into a recorder or camera. Get it out through words or journaling. Write it down, word for word. Deal with every detail, no matter how painful, gut-wrenching or heart-rending. If the thoughts, words or statements are so uncomfortable that you don't want others to ever see what you've written, shred or burn immediately after getting it out. It's not about storing the information. It's about purging these stressors from your mind, body, spirit and life.

☐ **Laugh Until It Hurts** - Laughter is good medicine. Watch a comedy. Listen to a concert of your favorite comedian. Think back to the funniest thing you've ever seen or heard. Just laugh the heartiest of laughs. Try to find something to laugh about, all day, every day.

☐ **Just Breathe** - Taking deep breaths through the nose and breathing out the nose, twice as long as you inhaled, floods the cells with oxygen, which relieves stress.

I believe in attacking stress on many levels, with nutrition, behavior modification, supplements, homeopathy, exercise, sunshine and positive thinking. The health benefits that come with stress relief may well curb the spread of vitiligo and other diseases.

Since many vitiligo sufferers have noticed a correlation between their stress levels and their vitiligo becoming active, spreading or showing up for the first time, stress-reduction techniques are highly recommended for anyone fighting this disease.

A healthful personal life, surrounded by people you love and who love you is important. The compassion, human touch and opportunity to shed all pretentions and just be yourself, allowing every white spot to show without makeup or clothing or camouflage, may help you to become comfortable in your own (spotted) skin.

Chapter 3

Genetics, immune systems, vitiligo and other autoimmune diseases

Vitiligo is shown to have genetic and autoimmune origins. Whether you inherited vitiligo or your immune system went awry due to other factors, lifestyle is a key factor in determining whether genes, such as the ones that stimulate the onset of vitiligo, become active. Genetic health issues are shown to reverse with positive lifestyle changes.

The latest research points to several autoimmune diseases found in the gene pool of those suffering with generalized vitiligo. Vitiligo is most closely linked to Celiac disease and rheumatoid arthritis.

Other autoimmune diseases that are very closely linked to vitiligo include Type 1, or autoimmune diabetes, Grave's disease, multiple sclerosis and systemic lupus erythematosus.

Protein effecting lymph cells that may produce tumors and the enzymes effecting T and B cells that may terminate immune responses, as well as enzymes blocking the making of tyrosinase are also found in the gene pools of those with generalized vitiligo.

(Retrieved from Variant of *TYR* and Autoimmunity Susceptibility Loci in Generalized Vitiligo)

Since we've been dealt this blow of having an autoimmune disease and genetic disease, what can we do about it? Studies show changing to a healthful, active and happy lifestyle may do wonders for our health, despite the genetic link. We have the power to change our health, our lives, and our vitiligo!

More specifically, vitiligo and other autoimmune clients should focus heavily on a Celiac diet, removing all gluten foods. I recommend that anyone suffering from any autoimmune disease request testing for Celiac and other autoimmune diseases.

Gluten grains such as wheat, oats, barley, rye and others are dangerous foods for those who suffer with vitiligo and other autoimmune diseases, including those diagnosed with Celiac.

These gluten foods also have the potential of allergens, in addition to possibly raising acidic levels in the body. I recommend avoiding these grains or only consuming them sporadically, and in small amounts, if at all. Corn, though not a gluten grain, is a grain with high-allergy potential, and is therefore best avoided as well.

The only grain that I recommend eating on a consistent basis is organic brown rice, with organic wild rice, which is actually a grass, if not allergic to grasses.

I also encourage proper eating. I highly recommend eating as close to nature as possible, with organic, locally grown foods that are fresh and in season. Fruits that are raw, in season, organic and fresh, are recommended for breakfast. Fruit is a high-energy food that may help to jumpstart your day, while potentially helping to clear waste from the system.

Such fresh, in-season, raw and organic vegetables are recommended several times a day for snacks and meals. Vegetables contain minerals, vitamins, enzymes and are a low-calorie food that should be the main staple of meals. Nightshade vegetables such as tomatoes, eggplant, okra and bell peppers are best avoided when balancing the immune system for health.

One to 2 glasses of fresh water upon awakening may help to flush out toxins that have settled into the body overnight. A glass of water per hour during waking hours may help to ensure proper hydration, removal of waste and better functioning organs, glands, cells, lymph and blood.

With any health challenges, it is best to avoid genetically modified or engineered foods, also known as GMO foods. Eating organic is the safest and most effective way to avoid GMO foods.

With any autoimmune disease or concern, I encourage everyone to get tested for allergies. Allergies stress the immune system and may lead to chronic inflammation. Getting allergy shots, removing offending foods, resting properly, as well as stress reduction, may all help to ensure the immune system is not overtaxed, potentially making it easier to balance the immune system, in the quest to heal and balance the entire body, mind and spirit.

Finally, supplements may prove beneficial to balancing the immune system, as well as potentially relieving autoimmune issues such as vitiligo. Some supplements that I take to balance my immune system include an under-the-tongue protein supplement that is shown to help to balance the immune system. (Available at www.TheWellnessWell.net)

From age 3, the thymus begins to shrink. By the time we reach 50, the thymus has shrunk so much we are barely making thymic protein. This is so much a part of my daily routine for general health, immune health and vitiligo health, that I use up to 3 packets per day. The National Institutes of Health has determined that Thymic Protein A is a potent immunoregulator.

Thymus protein is shown to assist in reversing the effects of aging. It helps to prevent or shorten the length of colds and flu viruses and other illnesses, as well as helping the immune system fight off daily stressors, a topic we touched on in the previous chapter.

You may not have inherited the best set of genes; however, your lifestyle may well dictate whether the genetic pool helps or hurts your chances of a full, healthful life!

It is best to get annual physicals to ensure you keep abreast of your overall health, though vitiligo itself is not considered dangerous or life-threatening. The corresponding underlying and often hidden diseases may present other health challenges that go beyond the so-called cosmetic disease, vitiligo.

Chapter 4

Glandular health and its close link to vitiligo

People with vitiligo need to focus on glandular health. Thyroid health is so closely related to vitiligo, that vitiligo is considered a symptom of a malfunctioning thyroid. Ask your doctor to perform an Anti-thyroglobulin antibodies, TSH 3 and TSH 4, as well as free T3 and T4, and TPO.

(Retrieved from thyroid.about.com/od/gettestedanddiagnosed/a/bloodtests.htm.)

Broda Barnes self testing may give a baseline and is often used for sub-clinical thyroid dysfunction that may not show up on traditional tests. I highly recommend getting tested regularly for thyroid dysfunction with a qualified endocrinologist. Again, vitiligo and thyroid dysfunction are so intertwined that vitiligo is considered a symptom of a malfunctioning thyroid.

The thyroid is very important to vitiligo health as well as health in general. The thyroid controls every metabolic process in the body. Weight gain, cold hands and feet, hair loss, brain fog, low body temperature, lack of energy and inability to lose weight while regularly exercising are some of the symptoms associated with hypothyroidism. Hypothyroidism is closely linked to vitiligo, autoimmune diseases, degenerative diseases and aging.

Another aspect of immunity and vitiligo is other autoimmune issues that may coincide with vitiligo, or may be prevalent in the families of those with vitiligo.

In addition to hypothyroidism, other autoimmune diseases related to vitiligo include Addison's disease, pernicious anemia, alopecia, lupus, Celiac disease, rheumatoid arthritis, muscular sclerosis, polyglandular dysfunction and diabetes.

I recommend annual physicals to ensure you keep abreast of your overall health and requesting tests for all glandular function.

As I mentioned in a previous chapter, nourishing the adrenal glands is important to general health. Adrenal supplements may encourage a balanced immune system and lower stress-related damage that may contribute to the spread or onset of vitiligo.

Exhausted adrenals are shown to hinder health and healing, weaken immunity and could exacerbate the negative effects of autoimmune diseases such as vitiligo.

I highly recommend that anyone suffering from vitiligo educate himself or herself about the endocrine system and check for information on symptoms of malfunction.

Ultimately, we know ourselves best and are the best judges of whether something is "off."

Polyglandular dysfunction manifests as disease. Polyglandular failure-related diseases include pernicious anemia, type 1 diabetes and immune mediated diabetes, alopecia, Celiac disease, hypogonadism, sjogren syndrome, rheumatoid arthritis, gastric carcinoid tumor, pancreatic deficiency malabsorption and vitiligo.

Vitiligo is associated with many autoimmune endocrinopathies. Patients with an early age of onset are less likely to have PAS II or other endocrinopathies. (Retrieved from http://emedicine.medscape.com/article/124398-overview).

The pancreas is responsible for helping to metabolize carbohydrates and proteins.

The pancreas is the body's sewer system. It is where the wastes and broken down particles of what we eat are filtered. A broken down sewer is very bad news for health, just as sewage backing up in a house or septic tank bring all that nasty, smelly and putrid waste into areas where it doesn't belong.

I include the Raw Pancreas supplement with heavy meals, to aid in digesting proteins and carbohydrates, as well as to keep bodily waste flowing out of the system efficiently.

The pineal gland also may play a role in healthy skin pigment. This gland produces the hormone melatonin. I take melatonin nightly. It reduces sharply as we age. Melatonin is shown to encourage a restful sleep and is considered a powerful brain antioxidant.

Again, polyglandular failure is linked to vitiligo. I recommend nourishing all of the glands to potentially ward off vitiligo and other glandular-related diseases.

Raw glandulars that are meant to nourish and support the glands are available at www.TheWellnessWell.net.

Chapter 5

Digestion, metabolism, absorption and vitiligo

Vitiligo sufferers may have a sluggish metabolism. Hypothyroidism and low stomach acid are often associated with vitiligo, which directly effects digestion, metabolism and nutrient absorption. Some of the effects of a sluggish metabolism may include poor protein digestion, poor carbohydrate digestion, poor assimilation of nutrients, and of course, vitiligo itself.

Since the thyroid controls all metabolic processes, digestion is compromised when the thyroid is not working properly. To improve digestion, I use vegetable-based digestive enzymes, along with hydrochloric acid, which is shown lacking in vitiligo sufferers.

Liver congestion is also implicated in vitiligo. Many people who come down with hepatitis develop vitiligo as a side effect. Liver nourishment and cleansing are recommended.

I use and recommend freshly squeezed lemon on a tablespoon with olive oil nightly, which may improve liver health. There are herbals that are shown to help improve liver function as well.

Drinking pure mineral water with fresh squeezed lemon and warm lemon water are also recommended to improve liver health.

I highly recommend juicing for people who suffer with vitiligo or any other autoimmune disease, glandular imbalance or degenerative disease. Juicing predigests nutrients. Fresh juicing circumvents the digestive process, allowing the freshly squeezed nutrients to go directly into the bloodstream. It's like getting a shot of vitamins, minerals and live enzymes delivered immediately.

Please note that bottled juice does not contain the live enzymes in freshly squeezed juices. Shelf juices are no substitute for freshly squeezed juicing.

A potential liver-cleansing juice recipe that I highly recommend includes fresh beets – bulbs and leaves, fresh parsley, fresh dandelion greens, fresh fennel, carrots, apple or pear with a small amount of fresh ginger.

Two refreshing digestive aids that are enzyme powerhouses include fresh papaya and pineapple, after meals.

In addition to juicing, hemp protein smoothies are a part of my regimen. I use organic, unsweetened vanilla almond milk, hemp protein powder, a touch of agave and organic frozen strawberries, with a fresh organic banana, blended, to make a meal substitute or snack. The protein is predigested and easily assimilated.

Eating fresh fruits, vegetables and nuts, in their natural and unaltered state are very highly recommended. When these foods are fresh, organic, in season and locally grown, they are the optimum foods for our bodies. The climates and mineral makeup of the local environment closely resemble the mineral contents in our bodies, so these foods are best for us, in terms of assimilation, nutrients and pollens that we breathe and live with daily.

Diet is of utmost importance to general health, and is shown beneficial to counteracting the effects of genetics and autoimmunity. Since Celiac disease is one of the illnesses that is closely related to vitiligo, and is part of polyglandular failure, a gluten-free diet may help to lessen the stress and strain on the immune system, and hence, help to lessen the effects of vitiligo. I try to eat gluten-free all the time.

A macrobiotic type diet that consists of fresh vegetables, fruits, nuts and brown rice as the only grain may offer a good aid in absorption and digestive health.

This type of simple diet, rich in vegetables and nutritive foods that nourish, heal and build up the body, may help to lower inflammation, reduce allergens that may be hidden, and balance the immune system and repair a leaky gut.

Gluten foods such as wheat may produce subtle, hidden allergies that go unnoticed, producing inflammation that keeps the immune system in attack mode. Quelling or lowering these potential allergens may help to calm and balance the immune system. The immune system attacking itself in various ways, such as deactivating melanocytes, is what happens to the skin of vitiligo sufferers. Anything we can do to lower or stop these immune system attacks will likely benefit vitiligo.

Low stomach acid in vitiligo sufferers is linked to low intrinsic factor, which may lead to B12 deficiency, often found in vitiligo sufferers, as well as pernicious anemia, which is closely related to vitiligo. Addison's disease is also a concern in the inability to absorb vitamin B12.

B12 injections are shown helpful in vitiligo, Addison's disease and pernicious anemia; however, there is some doubt as to whether sublingual B12 or oral doses of B12 are beneficial at all. Nasal B12 is said to be beneficial, when rubbed into the mucous membranes of the nose, using a Q-tip application.

I recommend B12 shots if your doctor feels they are necessary, as well as NOW brand Instant Energy B12 packets daily.

Other B vitamins, such as PABA, folic acid, phenylalanine and B6 are lacking in many vitiligo sufferers, so a daily supplement of all B vitamins is recommended. Further, research shows that extra vitamin C, vitamin D3, zinc and amino acids such as tyrosine, may drastically improve the health and condition in vitiligo sufferers. A multiple vitamin/mineral supplement that contains all of these nutrients is recommended daily.

To further aid in absorption of minerals, sea minerals are recommended, in water, as part of the daily regimen. Our blood is perfectly matched to the mineral content in sea water. We can actually get a sea water blood transfusion, when blood isn't available. I also take homeopathic bio plasma as part of my daily regimen, to ensure proper mineral ratio in my body.

To ensure I'm getting all the vitamins, minerals and nutrients I need to balance my system and help my vitiligo, I use a multiple vitamin and mineral supplement, extra vitamin C, vitamin D3 and liquid amino acids, in addition to the Hemp protein shakes that are rich in Omega 3 fatty acids as well as amino acids, in the form of powdered protein.

Omega 3 fatty acids are sorely lacking in modern diets. I eat a diet rich in Omega 3 wild fish, with the skin left on, such as salmon, sardines, mackerel and herring. It is important to leave the skin on fish to reap the benefits of the Omega 3 fatty acids. I also eat other Omega 3-rich foods, such as chia, hemp, black seed oil capsules, krill oil capsules and wild fish oil capsules.

Omega 3 fatty acids show anti-inflammatory benefits and support general health of mind, body and spirit.

One of the other ways that I encourage a potentially balanced digestive system is drinking bottled still mineral water, which potentially nourishes the cells, aids in circulation of blood and lymph, flushes organs and hydrates the system. Water is useful in potentially pushing toxins out of the body and is seen as the most important first aid in traditional naturopathy.

Adding minerals to distilled or filtered water is an option to increase the amount of mineral rich, pure water consumed daily. Adequate water intake is necessary for proper glandular function.

Leaky Gut Syndrome is often implicated when it comes to malabsorption. A fresh, whole foods and gluten-free diet, fresh water, digestive aids such as fermented foods and drinks, aloe vera juice, and reducing stress may aid in healing a leaky gut.

Wine is a raw, fermented alcoholic beverage, and the only alcohol I recommend for health. Organic red wine has so many potential benefits to health, I highly recommend a glass with dinner.

Other fermented foods that are potentially healthful include fermented cabbage, which is easy to make. The billions of beneficial bacteria are well worth the efforts.

I take a head of cabbage and shred it, after thoroughly cleaning it. I place it in a glass dish with distilled water, a small amount of apple cider vinegar and a glass top. It sits on the counter for 3 to 4 days, fermenting, before I begin using it as a side dish and drinking its juice.

Some of the other potentially beneficial fermented foods include coconut kefir drinks, acidophilus, apple cider vinegar, red wine vinegar and olives.

Recipes that call for milk are easily replaced with plain kefir. Also, flavored kefir as a breakfast drink substitute, or mixed with raw, gluten-free granola, makes a great meal. Kefir is a good dessert starter.

Think about what you consume, for you are what you eat; but more importantly, you are what you absorb. Choosing foods and supplements for their health benefits, easy absorption, gut healing and digestion promoting properties, should be foremost on your minds.

Avoiding pre-packaged foods, gluten foods, sugar, dyes and additives, may take some of the stress and strain off of organs, and may promote healthful digestion, absorption and metabolizing of nutrients.

Gluten foods include wheat, rye, barley and oats. Breads, pastas, crackers, oatmeal, cookies, cakes and pies made with gluten may cause autoimmune diseases such as vitiligo to worsen.

The recommended diet is rich in live, fresh foods. A diet that is highly alkaline or acid reducing is best. Too much acidity in the blood is a symptom of too little acid in the stomach. A whole foods-based healthful diet is shown to help balance alkalinity to acid in the body; thus promoting potentially perfect health.

It is important to note that lemons and other acidic fruits help to promote stomach acid; therefore, these foods help to promote alkaline blood. In other words, acid for the stomach is very different than acid in the blood, which is dangerous when it overwhelms the alkaline to acid ratio.

Though citrus, vinegar, and Vitamin C are high in acid, they are actually good for our bodies, helping to aid digestion, and thereby allowing a healthful alkaline-based blood – the fluid of life.

Acidic foods like lemons actually leave an alkaline footprint when burned to ash; therefore citrus is an alkaline food.

Beyond stevia, the one sweetener that I recommend is agave, made from the agave plant. This sweetener has a low glycemic index, as well as prebiotics FOS and inulin, which are necessary for digestive health.

Agave often gets a bad rap, for there were corn syrup-type products that were called agave, but they were not made from the agave plant. Many holistic consultants still have the misconception that pure agave nectar is somehow a corn syrup product. It is not. Further, there is a movement that is comparing agave's inulin and FOS to high fructose corn syrup in its dangers to health. The evidence is not there to support this.

High fructose corn syrup is really a misnomer, since the syrups are mostly glucose, with very little fructose, or fruit sugar present.

Agave and stevia are two sweeteners shown to improve health, promote beneficial gut bacteria and aid in proper digestion.

Eating meals in a stress-free, relaxing environment is highly recommended. Rushing to eat, eating while watching television or while working on the computer, eating while upset, or in stress-inducing situations, are potentially harmful to digestion and are highly discouraged.

A beautiful dining room, fine china, flowers, naturally based and scented candles, good company with festive and positive conversation, are a good example of a productive meal-consuming environment.

A glass of raw, fermented organic red wine or a warm cup of mint tea may be the perfect end to a perfect meal! Cheers!

Chapter 6

Feed and nourish your skin naturally

The skin is the body's largest organ. Most people don't think of the skin as a means of absorbing nutrients; however, it is just that! Remember, more important than *you are what you eat* is that *you are what you absorb!*

Taking care of your skin the way that you take care of the inside of your body is of utmost importance to skin health, and potentially healing to vitiligo.

I try to avoid soaps and other skin products that have artificial dyes, colors, perfumes and harsh chemicals. I try to use brands that are healthful, and use the same ingredients that I feel comfortable ingesting.

There are all natural soaps, lotions, bubble baths and other skin products that are nutrient rich and healthful.

Essential oils such as peppermint, lavender, bergamot, lemon grass, nut oils, olive oil, and many healthful and natural ingredients that potentially help to heal the skin from the outside inward, are ones to look for in products to use on the skin and on vitiligo.

Vitamins that are near expiration are an excellent choice for a vitamin bath. Crushing vitamins and other supplement tablets or capsules for use in the bath, along with an aloe vera-based bubble bath and seaweed powder, is one of my favorite skin-nourishing baths.

Detoxifying baths are potentially healthful and nourishing to the skin. I really like the alkalizing baths that include baking soda, Epsom salts, sea salt and lavender oil, at night, as warm as I can stand it, with the jets on to relax and potentially pull out toxins through my largest organ – the skin.

Body scrubs are another healthful way to remove debris, old skin, and potentially encourage toxin removal through the skin. I like to mix coarse sea salt, coconut oil or castor oil, bayberry oil, black pepper, ground into powder, beeswax, black seed powder, apple cider vinegar and liquid vitamins near expiration, rubbed onto the skin. These healing nutrients leave the skin soft, supple and ready to absorb nutrient-rich Vitiligo Herbal Skin Cream that is available at www.TheWellnessWell.net

I have actually taken vitamin A capsules, along with other vitamins and supplements, and rubbed them directly on my vitiligo patches, with success in encouraging a freckle or two. Recycle those old vitamins, minerals and herbs to make a great nourishing bathing brew for healthful, glowing skin.

I have some loose teas that I've collected over the years. I often add some to a small sachet and hang it on the faucet as the water runs for my bath. Taking a tea bath infuses live enzymes, volatile oils and nutritive healing vitamins and minerals into my baths. Circumventing my digestive system and taking nutrients directly through the skin is a practice I've done for many years. I recommend it in clients with vitiligo or any illness.

One consistent compliment that I receive is the glowing, healthful look of my skin, despite my battle with vitiligo. Taking care of the skin, inside and outside, is part of my daily regimen. Younger, wrinkle-reduced skin is one of the potential payoffs of this ritual.

When brewing a pot of tea, any unused tea left in the pot is a good addition to the nightly bath, or a good addition to the homemade scrub.

A clay mask for the skin is also a part of my regimen. I sometimes make a mask using dry terramin clay, aloe vera juice, and a little calendula oil. I rub this mixture onto clean skin. I allow it to dry before showering it off or using a scrub to remove the clay. The clay is very absorbing and potentially draws toxins out of the skin.

Detoxifying the skin has many benefits, including relaxing the body, mind and spirit, as well as cleansing the body from the inside out, by pulling toxins through the skin. Just as sweat is a natural way of removing toxins through the skin, detoxifying baths potentially pull toxins away. The least amount of toxins built up in the system, the more efficient the system is able to balance and nourish the body, creating an environment whereby the body may heal itself.

Remember to love and nourish your skin with the same healthful ingredients that you put into your mouth for health. Skin is a breathing, absorbing organ that is a major detoxifying outlet of the body as well.

I recommend bathing with the honey and black seed soap, bath wash and lotion that are available at www.TheWellnessWell.net.

After my nightly baths, I leave my body moist as I apply Vitiligo Herbal Skin Cream to all of my patches, lighter-skinned areas and surrounding skin. Cells heal and repair at night as we sleep, so I've found this to be the best time to apply Vitiligo Herbal Skin Cream.

When I go biking or walking in the mornings, I try to apply Vitiligo Herbal Skin Cream to my vitiligo spots to encourage pigment in the healing sun.

This is one of the most effective tools I've used in my quest to regain my color. I'm very blessed that my vitiligo is not visible to most people.

Thanks to all the knowledge I'm sharing in this book, my color is returning to vitiligo patches daily!

This regimen and routine are one of the most important rituals in returning color to my vitiligo-inflicted skin. **Vitiligo Herbal Skin Cream** Extra Strength, that I customized to include many of the recommendations for re-pigmenting skin are available at www.TheWellnessWell.net.

Vitiligo Herbal Skin Cream contains the most active herbs that are directly shown to help re-pigment vitiligo on the market currently.

Up to 30 minutes of sunshine is recommended.

Moderate amounts of sunshine are shown beneficial to vitiligo sufferers.

Chapter 7

Detoxify your body

Detoxifying and cleaning the body internally, externally and through our diets and habits are shown to have a profoundly positive effect on our bodies and diseases, including vitiligo.

There are many detoxification programs. I try to use several at different stages during the year. We've touched on detoxifying with juicing, how we eat, how we improve digestion, through skin detoxifying baths and scrubs and other methods.

Now, we will focus on specific detoxifying cleanses that could benefit the body and facilitate healing vitiligo.

The vitamin C flush is a Detox that I believe is extremely beneficial to me and my quest for ultimate health and living a vitiligo-free life.

I like to have a celebratory setting around this cleanse. I get out a beautiful crystal pitcher and a crystal glass to partake of this potentially healing nectar.

I mix a heaping tablespoon of powdered ascorbate C, a flat tablespoon of powdered stevia, a flat tablespoon of pure B grade maple syrup, (its sediment is rich in B vitamins, minerals and enzymes), 3 Emergen-C packets Acai Berry flavored, a freshly squeezed organic lemon. Then I place the lemon halves into the pitcher, so that lemon oil will become a part of this C flush.

I try to drink a glass or more per hour. Some of the benefits I've noticed in doing this for a day or two include a thorough cleansing of my colon, clearing up congestion, headaches go away and sinus problems disappear. I also notice an energy surge when using the C flush. Sometimes, there is die off; however working through the healing crisis and staying on this cleanse has proven most beneficial for me. This is a detoxifying cleanse that I try to incorporate weekly since extra vitamin C is shown helpful to those with vitiligo.

Some of the reported benefits of a vitamin C flush include flushing out parasites, Candida and other fungi, bacteria and mucous. Clearing these health-degenerating problems from the digestive tract may also aid absorption. All health related problems that are shown to have a correlation to vitiligo and other diseases may benefit from a vitamin C flush.

Another detoxifying cleanse is the gluten-free diet, as stated before. This is a diet that I highly recommend as a lifestyle change. This detoxifying diet includes healthful Omega 3-rich fish, if not allergic, brown rice, fresh fruits, vegetables and raw, unsalted nuts, except for peanuts, which are linked to allergies and a potentially cancerous fungus. I especially recommend walnuts for their potential parasite-fighting properties, as well as the reported benefits of eating walnuts to those suffering with vitiligo and other diseases.

I highly recommend humus several times a week, as part of this detoxifying diet/lifestyle change. Some studies have shown that humus is beneficial to healing vitiligo.

Brown rice is the only grain recommended when detoxifying. It is important to note that vegetables are carbohydrates, so this is not a diet or lifestyle change to confuse with a low-carbohydrate diet.

Avoiding sugar, artificial sweeteners, canned foods, processed foods, preservatives and other chemicals are a mandatory part of this healing, detoxifying diet, that I recommend as a lifestyle change. If you want to live, eat live foods!

Spices such as cayenne, garlic, onions, ginger, cinnamon, fennel, black pepper, turmeric and other natural spices can be beneficial to vitiligo and are encouraged.

Vegetables and fruits are complex carbohydrates that are nourishing and healthful.

Fresh vegetables are the staple of this diet, in many colors, shapes and varieties; though I discourage the use of nightshade vegetables, such as tomatoes, okra, eggplant and bell peppers in all colors. These foods may cause allergic reactions, which are believed to promote inflammation.

Healing broths made with vegetables such as leeks, carrots, cabbage, root vegetables and other healthful foods, are highly recommended during this detoxifying cleanse/lifestyle change.

Again, experiment with vegetables, nuts, fruits and brown rice to create healthful recipes that keep these foods fresh and interesting, so that they become part of an overall lifestyle change of living a sugar-, chemical- and gluten-free life!

I encourage daily detoxifying of the body and not just an annual or semi-annual cleanse.

We need to keep our bodies clean and running efficiently all the time.

Prevention is key. A well-oiled machine, in this case, our bodies, is best equipped to run efficiently and correct itself.

Later this year, look for *Wanakee's Deliciously Divine Gluten – Free Cookbook*, for recipes that may help to facilitate this detoxifying lifestyle change.

10 Day Detoxifying Diet Plan

By Wanakee Hill, ND

To help get you started on a lifestyle changing detoxifying regimen, I'm including a bonus copy of my 10 day detoxifying diet plan.

I have devised a 10-day plan that may aid the body in clearing out stagnant matter that may lead to weight loss, lessening inflammation, removing excess water weight, boosting mental clarity, removing parasites, and raising energy levels and encouraging fat-burning.

I recommend starting the day, or 'breaking the fast,' with 2 glasses of water upon awakening, which may wash away toxins and debris that built up overnight. I further recommend fresh, ripe and in-season fruits, as the first meal of the day. Fresh fruit is shown to increase metabolism and release wastes from the body.

A mid-morning meal is usually a power shake that is stocked with Omega 3 fatty acids, which may feed the brain and nourish the entire body; helping to create a balanced ratio of Omega 3 fatty acids to our over abundance of Omega 6 fatty acids. To correct the imbalance of Omega 3s to Omega 6s in the diet, some practitioners recommend consuming 10 times more Omega 3s than Omega 6s.

This diet plan avoids common allergens and foods that are suspected in allergies as well as potentially acid-producing foods. There are some foods that I recommend banning permanently from the diet, including high-fructose corn syrup, trans-fatty acids, hydrogenated processed foods, most fast foods, artificial food dyes, colors and preservatives, as well as all artificial sweeteners.

This plan is specifically designed to include low-glycemic foods, avoiding typically offending foods such as meat, dairy, wheat, corn, peanuts and soy.

This diet plan is rich in Omega 3-enhancing foods such as wild, cold water fatty fish, vegetables, most nuts, fruits and berries. All of these are stone-age, hunter/gatherer foods that our ancestors ate. Nature based foods that our bodies are adept at consuming. The modern diets many of us have adopted have potentially led to many of the diseases, weight gain, chronic inflammation and accelerated aging that are so prevalent today. Though our diets have evolved, our brains, bodies and spirits are still more in tune with Omega 3-rich Paleolithic diets.

Our ratio of Omega 6 fatty acids that are found in high abundance in modern diets, and relatively low ratio of Omega 3 fatty acids found in today's foods, are literally creating physical and mental illnesses such as autoimmune and degenerative diseases.

It's time to get back to basics. Eating directly from a tree or garden, picking berries and other seeds from nature's pantry, is a healthful way to live and thrive.

Adopting this 10-day plan may ease depression, reduce inflammation that signals disease and malfunction in the body, nourish the cells and expel toxins and parasites, which lead to water retention, health problems, weight gain and autoimmune diseases.

It is important to include meditation and some form of exercise daily, to ensure the holistic being is covered from the mental, spiritual and physical aspects of your being.

Closing your eyes and deep breathing for 5 to 10 minutes per day are shown to help lower blood pressure, reduce stress and lead to a healthier life.

Savor the meals and foods that are recommended for the 10 days on the plan. I usually drink a cup of detoxifying dieter's tea right after dinner. The tea includes senna, to help cleanse the bowels, chickweed to reduce and metabolize body fat, black walnut leaf, which is a potential parasite remover and is rich in essential fatty acids, as well as licorice that is said to protect damaged and inflamed tissues. (Available at www.TheWellnessWell.net)

I recommend that you drink plenty of pure mineral-rich water during this 10-day plan to flush out toxins.

Please be sure to keep a diary of what you eat and how you feel. Email me with any concerns or comments at Wanakee@TheWellnessWell.net

The diet plan is very simple. Brown rice, most vegetables, (except nightshade), fruits and nuts, (except peanuts), are unlimited, though I do recommend eating fruits separately, for breakfast. Again, agave and stevia are the only recommended sweeteners, with B grade maple syrup during the Vitamin c flush.

Fish is recommended daily, including wild salmon, mackerel, herring and sardines. Baked, broiled or grilled, with a salad and dressing made with fresh olive oil, lemons and garlic, with cayenne, along with steamed, roasted or grilled vegetables in unlimited quantities. I recommend removing all breads or other simple carbohydrates, refined sugars and grains.

Vegetable broth made with onions, garlic, green, red and orange vegetables of your choice are boiled for 30 minutes. Strain liquid and use this broth every hour as nourishment and healing for two to three days.

I recommend eating sweet potatoes, cabbage, broccoli and cauliflower, as well as greens that are fresh, locally grown and in season.

Eight to 10 glasses of water are recommended daily, to target fats and toxins lingering in your body.

This gluten-free, nutrient-dense, Omega 3-rich diet could remove up to 10 pounds of fat and waste in a week, while reducing inflammation and helping to balance the immune system.

For more tips and recipes, join TheWellnessWell on Twitter and check out the blog on The Wellness Well web site.

Coming later this year:

Wanakee's Deliciously Divine

Gluten – Free Cookbook

Wanakee's vitiligo healing broth

Fresh vegetables from your garden or farmer's market

Boil these vegetables for 30 minutes.

Strain and refrigerate unused liquid portion.

Blend all vegetables in a food processor and freeze to use as a soup or bean thickener, as needed.

Warm a cup of broth daily, on a conventional stove.

No microwaving.

Organic and locally grown:

Radishes, bulbs and leaves

Ginger bulb

Mustard seeds

Pepper corns

Celery

Chickpeas

Seaweed flakes or strips

A dash of turmeric

Strain and drink with a dash of Amino Acids or add miso paste.

Chapter 8

Kee's Health Tips ©

A dozen health improvement tips

1. A gallon of extra virgin olive oil. Place 10 peeled garlic cloves in the bottle, along with 3 red chili peppers (fresh or dried). Allow to sit a few days, and then use it to cook, to season vegetables and popcorn or on anything for which you would use olive oil or butter. This is an excellent way to keep your heart and entire cardiovascular system tuned and nourished.
2. Consider eating the white membrane inside the rind of citrus fruit. It's loaded with disease-fighting phytonutrients. My mom knew this long before science recently started exploring the subject.
3. Dulse and kelp seaweed seasonings in a shaker. Use this as a substitute for salt on any and everything. Its sea salt content will give you the nourishing minerals you need, while your thyroid and entire system will benefit from the unlimited nutrients from sea vegetables in a simple and easy way.

4. Fresh fruits and vegetables that are in season and freshly picked locally and grown organically. A farmer's market near your home is the best place to buy vegetables. A better idea is to grow your own. These are the most nutrient-packed foods and will give the body what it needs to balance and heal itself.

5. Organic miso paste in a cup of hot water, as soup, once a day, for healing, nourishing and longevity. This fermented version of soy is the only soy that I recommend. Use in moderation.

6. An apple or pear a day, with the skin on and hopefully with a bit of stem. I eat the stem, for tree bark is very healthful and the fiber is good for your digestive system. I eat the seeds as well. Apple seeds have a minute amount of cyanide. Just enough to be helpful to our bodies, killing pathogens that may potentially harm us.

7. Bitter greens in a salad, juice and cooked with other foods nourish the body from head to toe and cleanse the liver and gallbladder.

8. Shredded cabbage, placed in an airtight bowl, completely covered with distilled water, apple cider vinegar and a dash of amino acids are a potential powerhouse of beneficial bacteria.

Allow it to ferment for a few days, then drink the juice and use the cabbage with some of the seasoned olive oil, walnuts and kalamata olive as a side dish. This fermented cabbage contains billions of beneficial bacteria and may help heal ulcers and give the digestive system a healing boost.

9. Eating sprouts. Sunflower sprouts are packed with protein, vitamins, minerals, enzymes and other life-giving properties. Alfalfa sprouts, mung bean sprouts and other sprouts, added to miso soup or a daily salad will give your body the healing energy it needs and deserves.

10. Reducing stress in your life. Getting rid of all stressors that you have the control to remove and doing healing meditation, yoga, brisk walks and stretching with breathing, with the intent to remove stress from your life.

11. Water, water, everywhere. Drinking water. Bathing in water. Using cold water as first aid. Water is a life-flowing force that is important to health and the staple of naturopathy!

12. Supplements are important to healing, since we likely never get the full spectrum of nutrients from our diets. Supplement for health!

Chapter 9

Herbal supplements that are shown to benefit vitiligo

Vitiligo herbal *picrorhiza* is shown to aid digestion and detoxify daily. Taken with dinner, *picrorhiza* is shown to:

- aid in digesting and metabolizing foods properly
- aid in halting the spread of vitiligo
- aid in raising immune boosting B cells and T cells
- aid in reducing the size and number of vitiligo patches
- aid in lowering inflammation
- aid in overall healing and disease prevention
- aid in liver cleansing and detoxifying

A recent study on Gingko Biloba suggested 400 mgs of Ginkgo given several times a day, helped to halt the spreading of vitiligo.

I don't take the 1200 mg of Ginkgo daily as recommended and used in the study; however, I do include ginkgo biloba in my daily supplement regimen.

I tend to stagger my supplements throughout the day. I take some before breakfast, some between breakfast and lunch, some before and after dinner, using others at bedtime.

I tend to take my raw thyroid supplement, raw adrenal cortex, raw pancreas and homeopathic supplements upon awaking, on an empty stomach.

I drink a cup of warm herbal tea and fresh mineral water upon awaking as well.

I then eat a fresh piece of fruit to energize my body and potentially help to flush out toxins and debris that have settled in overnight.

Later in the morning, I add an iodine supplement to nourish my thyroid further, as well as gingko, krill oil or hemp oil Omega 3. These are all potentially healing to vitiligo and an important part of my supplement regimen. I also have a small glass of coconut kefir to ensure beneficial bacteria in my intestinal flora, as well as supplementing with acidophilus.

After lunch, I tend to take enzyme therapy capsules that include hydrochloric acid, pepsin and bitters. I make a potentially healing salad dressing that includes red wine vinegar, oil and agave. I also take an herbal fat burner to facilitate my metabolism and increase energy.

I try to have a cup of tea and a glass of water hourly, during the day, to ensure proper hydration, so that my body fluids are moving freely, getting oxygen to the cells and removing toxins from the body.

Later in the day, I may have hemp oil capsules, or chia oil capsules, to ensure Omega 3 fatty acids are prevalent in my body.

I usually have some kind of wild fish, at least once a day, plenty of salads and other vegetable-rich meals, which also infuse potentially healing nutritional boosts throughout the day.

Herbs such as stinging nettle and Chinese chlorella are helpful supplements. These herbs are some of the few vegetable-based sources of vitamin B 12. I also try to take a ginseng vial, as well as royal jelly/bee pollen supplements toward evening.

Up to three times a day, I take Pro Boost Thymic A protein powder packets, under my tongue. Thymic Protein A has proven invaluable in my quest for health. The thymus is no longer producing much Thymic Protein A by age 50, and those with immune dysfunction may benefit greatly from the immune system balancer. I have noticed that it seems to help grow my hair and I also believe it helps to stimulate pigment in my vitiligo patches. I recommend this supplement for anyone suffering with immune issues or anyone past the age of 40. It is available at www.TheWellnessWell.net.

I believe that allergies are a major threat to immune health. Not only do allergies cause uncomfortable to painful symptoms, allergies also create harmful inflammation. I got tested for allergies and began allergy shots. My quality of life has improved drastically since I started these shots.

Allergy shots are a gradual buildup of allergic properties, which are introduced in small amounts that are increased over time. This method encourages the immune system to build up a tolerance to offending substances, so that the immune system is not constantly fighting these allergens, and thus undermining the strength and resources of immune responses.

As I age, my body reminds me that my thymus has shrunk and I can no longer tolerate certain things, including gardening outside, for my allergies have progressed with age. Understanding how the body loses immune-fighting ability, through the loss of Thymic Protein A, along with constantly fighting autoimmunity, and the underlying inflammation that goes along with allergens, I am better equipped to work toward correcting the imbalances, rather than using medications to mask the symptoms, which may bring only temporary relief.

Daily sunshine is a supplement that we all should strive to get, research shows. Even if the sun is hidden behind clouds or if it's cold, a half hour of early morning sun may potentially aid in healing vitiligo, providing vitamin D3, shown low or lacking in many vitiligo sufferers, raising mood and providing many other life-giving properties to the body, mind and spirit. I consider sunshine as essential to my health and well-being as any nutrient that I must have to live.

At some point during the day, I try to take Sam-E, separate from other nutrients and on an empty stomach. Sam-E has anti-inflammatory properties and is valuable in potentially ridding my body of vitiligo and dysfunction.

At night, I attempt to nourish my pineal gland with melatonin supplements as well as 5HTP. Replacing what the body is lacking encourages balance and health, I believe. I try to provide the natural tools necessary to ensure my body is equipped to fight off anything that may prove dangerous to my body, health, mind or well-being. I often use the Auyervedic herb,

Triphala, at night, to help with digestion, absorption and ultimately good gut health.

Fighting vitiligo is a job that is best attacked with nutrition, inside and outside, I firmly believe. This method has proven most effective for me.

The same theory of taking care of your car is true of taking care of your body. Preventive maintenance is far better than paying for repairs due to neglect.

There are many other herbals that I have tried over the years. Some were too expensive to continue. Others did not have the benefits that I was looking for, in a reasonable amount of time.

I have found it is best to evolve. I listen to my body, try to give it what it needs and try to stay as close to nature as possible, in my quest for healing.

I often say to clients, our bodies are not made up of chemicals. We are nutrient-run machines. The cleaner and purer the nutrients that we put into our bodies, the better the chance of a balanced body that can and potentially will repair and heal itself.

Through research, talking to many people who are going through the same trials that I'm facing, and working with my own body, I've learned to accept the changes in my body, while working to correct or prevent deficiencies so that my problems do not overtake my body.

I strive to replace the important things that are missing, to encourage a well balanced and well functioning body, at any age.

I have no fear of aging, nor do I believe that vitiligo is hopeless. I do believe that I am conquering this disease with a steady progression toward perfect balance and potentially, perfect health. You can too!

Chapter 10

An overview

The pep talk!

In conclusion, I wrote this book to educate on the role of Celiac disease, faulty digestion, glandular imbalance, genetics and other factors that are shown to have a role in vitiligo. I stress the importance of how correcting these problems may halt the spread of vitiligo and eventually encourage our bodies to repair and restore. Those who are suffering with other autoimmune or degenerative diseases, this holistic healing approach is shown to potentially improve your health and ability to heal. For those of you who are members of **The Wellness Well** online support group and members of **VSIG**, you are likely familiar with some of this information.

VSIG is an alternative healing support group for people with vitiligo. Most of us were told our disease is "incurable" and there is nothing we can do about it. Prevailing wisdom has said, it is harmless and will not kill you. Pioneers who sought to find a cause explored the possibility of digestive problems -- malabsorption, low stomach acid, liver problems, vitamin and mineral deficiencies, glandular imbalances, strained emotions and stress. We, in turn, explored ways to improve these conditions with food, herbs, rest and water. Follow Vitiligo VSIG on Facebook.

People with vitiligo know the debilitating emotional pain that comes with helplessness when told there is no cure. We know the anguish of not knowing when or if the colorless patches will spread. Vitiligo sufferers know the discomfort when people stare at the white lesions that spot our skin in such a horrid way or ask if you have AIDS, as many in Africa are routinely asked. The pain of wanting to be normal, whole, healed and healthy is often alleviated through education and support groups. Please join our **VSIG** support group blog: www.TheWellnessWell.net

Many of us have defied the odds. Through research, information sharing and our own unscientific trials, we've made many discoveries about our vitiligo, our health and the dysfunctions that science now validates. We've become comfortable in our own skin, as we understand the underlying nutritional, glandular and gut dysfunction that seem to go hand in hand with vitiligo. We have learned acceptance and power in educating ourselves and taking control of our own health, in a naturally holistic way.

We have discovered many commonalities, such as a sluggish metabolism, thyroid dysfunction, liver congestion, symptoms consistent with Leaky Gut Syndrome, poor absorption of proteins, depression, B vitamin deficiencies, including B12, B6, PABA, and folic acid that research has shown plague most, if not all of us. We now have evidence that Celiac disease, or gluten intolerance may well play a very large roll in these maladies, as well as its very close genetic association to vitiligo.

We have noticed many of us are high strung and have a lot of stress in our lives that often precedes vitiligo onset or spreading. We've also found there's usually some family history of thyroid problems, early graying, alopecia, allergies, diabetes and other autoimmune ailments in our own lives or the lives of relatives.

Luckily, there have been naturally oriented doctors who have done experiments on using B12 shots, PABA shots, and other vitamin therapies, with success. These doctors have given us a glimpse into the things that are wrong in our bodies and how correcting these things may bring about positive change in restoring color to our skin.

By most accounts, one prevailing theory among those of us who have researched and lived with the disease, as well as naturally oriented practitioners, is that vitiligo is a disease of malnutrition. No, we're not starving or in any way food-deprived. We are, however, shown lacking the digestive health and balance to absorb some nutrients through our diets and current health status, until we begin to actively change our lifestyles to promote digestive health.

This book addresses the issues that we have through nutrition. We focus on the healing powers of water – drinking it, bathing in it, making it an important part of our nutritional quest for optimum digestion and health. Do you keep track of the amount of water you drink each day? I recommend water with fresh lemon throughout the day to potentially help liver function. It not only gives the water flavor, it adds the extra digestive friendly boost of acid to the stomach.

Make your food appealing. The ritual of preparing the nutrients should be festive and happy. When we like the way our food and drink look, we are more apt to partake in a satisfying, gut-appeasing way.

I hope that this book becomes a blueprint to a happier, healthier body and digestive tract that may help you avoid illness and correct imbalances in your bodies.

Whatever disease or illness you're battling or want to prevent, a healthful, holistic lifestyle is your best potential defense.

Hopefully, you sleep well nightly. A full 8 hours is recommended. You awaken. It's morning. It's time to break the fast, or eat breakfast. I recommend fresh fruit. A peach, a banana, a plum, grapes, cherries, watermelon or something fresh, in season and organic, to start the day. Fruit, like water, has potentially cleansing abilities. It helps to wash away old cellular debris and it starts the trek through the digestive cycle pushing waste through the colon. Enzymes are of utmost importance to digestion. One of the best ways to ensure our bodies get live enzymes is to eat live foods, in their raw state. No better time to give the body nature's perfect food than in the morning. Fruit, in the morning is a perfect start to every perfect day!

After my morning shower on weekends, I hope to find my husband making buckwheat pancakes, a rare gluten-free treat, indeed. If I'm not so lucky, I make a protein shake. My favorite protein shakes include either brown rice protein or hemp protein, with almond milk, a bit of agave to sweeten and organic frozen strawberries, fresh banana and a noisy blender. This is a delicious, filling and complete breakfast. It gives me the fiber I need, along with protein, vitamins, minerals and enzymes, to ensure my day starts off right.

My husband often gets a hardy workout. When I tag along, we usually bike for half an hour, before heading to the neighborhood pool, when the weather permits. In the pool, we march, step, twist, turn and basically, give our bodies a great aerobic-resistant training workout. It's a lot of fun, and we dry our bodies in the sun and wind on our bike ride back home. This movement is such fun, it's almost weird calling it exercise, but it is a workout. Good digestion is aided by body movement. There is no specific movement that is mandatory. Just move. If you like to dance, play the music as you go about your household chores. Dance with the mop. Waltz with the broom! Just move! Moving is an important way to get lymph fluids moving. It is of utmost importance to move the lymph fluids for perfect health and balance. Movement is also important to mental health, releasing endorphins or happy hormones. Sunshine is shown to lift the mood as well. Many consider vitiligo a disease of mental health and stress.

Got pets? These companions do wonders for our stress levels. Taking the family pooch for a stroll after a meal helps to digest foods. Pets are such loyal family members and studies show they reduce our stress levels. Stress reduction is extremely important to digestive health and overall health. What are some of the ways you reduce stress? A koi pond is wonderful, for fish are said to lower stress as well as blood pressure.

It's a good idea to take a minute to relax, close your eyes and breathe. Take deep breaths in, deep breaths out as you think about beautiful tropical waters – calm, serene, relaxing. This is a form of meditation; a great relaxer and a great way to sooth your mind, body and digestive system. Meditation just before a meal allows our digestive systems to absorb the meal uninhibited. Tension, stress, emotional upheaval and anxiety are harmful to digestion and are best relieved before we take a bite of food.

Speaking of biting food, how thoroughly do you chew? Has anyone ever seen undigested chunks of food in the stool? Chewing slowly, methodically, and thoroughly until the food is liquid is the best way to ensure we get the nutrients into our systems. Eating too fast lessens digestion, forces the liver to work harder and robs us of the all important vitamins, minerals, enzymes and amino acids needed for health. By taking the time to really chew our food, we immediately improve our digestion in addition to really tasting the foods we eat.

Socialization and happy feelings also aid digestion. Sitting too long encourages a sluggish system. Stretch your legs reach out your hand and enjoy human contact.

When shopping for food, I try to emphasize fruits and vegetables, lean proteins, healthy fats, whole grain brown rice and legumes.

These are the healthful foods that potentially help your gut heal and encourage optimum nutrition. These are the foods that help to encourage an alkaline body. When you are a bit hungry between the smaller meals I hope you are eating, think about nuts! Yes, I know… every doctor, nurse and nutritionist in hospitals have said, nuts are fattening! What they fail to acknowledge, or perhaps, it's a failure of knowledge… nuts are good fats. We need essential fatty acids in our diets, especially Omega 3 fatty acids. Nuts, olives, olive oil, coconut oil, walnut oil, grapeseed oil, hemp oil, chia seeds and oil, are all great sources of good fats. I encourage keeping walnuts around at all times. Walnuts are not only a good source of fats; walnuts are potentially good for vitiligo. Some of the Africans in the VSIG support group have talked about people who drink a tea made of green walnut hulls daily, and have regained their pigment; some in about a year! Yes, walnuts are healthful in many ways. They are shown to rid the body of parasites that inhibit digestion. Enjoy the good fat in the walnuts and other fresh, raw and unsalted nuts.

Omega fatty acids are anti-inflammatory, feed the brain and are said to help with autoimmune diseases, of which vitiligo is classified. Ensuring Omega 3 rich oils are a part of your diet is one of the many ways to ensure your digestive juices are flowing in the right direction.

For lunch, I recommend vegetable salads that include baby greens of various types, fresh slices of avocado, sesame seeds, onions, carrots, radishes, and a freshly made garlic, olive oil and lemon dressing. Sardines or other high Omega 3 fish as a salad topper make this salad a hearty and healthful meal. All of the raw salad foods potentially aid digestion. This is a great meal to have for lunch daily. A big salad of live foods, chewed well, is a shot of nutrition to the gut! Complex carbohydrate rich salads add vitamins, minerals, enzymes and healing chlorophyll.

Salads, lean protein, good fats, and herbal seasonings like garlic and cayenne, help to protect you from constipation and add a real boost of fiber and nutrition to your daily lives. Check out all the colors and textures in a salad. Salads are vibrant and bursting with flavor. For those of you who have not acquired a taste for salad, make a concerted effort to enjoy the symphony of live foods. Your gut, health and waistline will certainly thank you, over and over and over again! For a nice healthful crunch, consider topping salads with raw nuts, except peanuts, which I do not recommend.

This is how I eat almost every day. I practice what I'm sharing. The diet and lifestyle that I'm putting forth in this book promotes an acid-alkaline balance that is absolutely essential to health, digestion and ridding the body of imbalances that lead to illnesses and disease.

Like everyone else, I like good food. I realize, however, that good food is whole food. Live food nourishes and enhances life. I hope this is a lifestyle change you're willing to make, starting now.

For a change of pace, a glass of sparkling mineral water with fresh squeezed pineapple juice is a champagne substitute you may have with special occasion meals. Make a toast, such as "to your health!" It will make your meal special and memorable. Even the children may partake. Pineapples are full of healthful enzymes that aid digestion. Mixing it with a sparkling mineral water gives us the sense of soda. Soda, with its phosphates, robs us of health and digestive balance. Your favorite naturally sweet fruit freshly squeezed in a juicer, then mixed with mineral water, is the perfect substitute for sodas. Fresh squeezed apples and ginger with a bit of agave and sparkling mineral water is a great ginger ale.

I have found that eliminating gluten from my diet has made me feel better and it seems to stimulate coloring in my vitiligo patches. The more digestion enhancing improvements I make to my body, the better the progress I'm noticing.

Brown rice, gluten free buckwheat for pancakes, along with quinoa- and amaranth-based pastas are recommended. Sometimes, I season the brown rice with garlic and seaweed flakes after it cooks, with olive oil. Other times, I use turmeric and saffron, to make yellow rice that is seasoned with seaweed flakes.

Fresh wild fish, with the skin on, for there is rich Omega 3 fatty acid in the skin. A meal with brown and wild rice as well as wilted bitter greens that include dandelion, turnip and mustard greens is delectable and easy to prepare. These bitter greens, as well as the turmeric in the brown rice, are music to your liver. Bitters aid digestion and are shown to ease the pressure on of the liver.

These foods are based on macrobiotic principles and are highly recommended to potentially reduce inflammation-causing problems in the body. A happy liver is imperative to balanced digestion.

Before eating, it's a good idea to pause and think about the bountiful meal you are about to enjoy. Think about the local growers who produced these foods without pesticides and hormones. Reflect on the icy waters of the Pacific Ocean, where wild salmon spun before gracing tables. The beautiful herbs that were freshly grown to season our foods and their wonderful smells are evident, when we stop to appreciate what is put before us. As you partake of meals, take deep breaths between bites. Feel the energy, extra nutrients and dense power of the food you are chewing slowly. Locally and organically grown foods are much more nutrient-dense than the foods in the market, shipped from other states or other countries. No wax. No pesticides. No processing. Foods the way nature intended. Embrace every bite for its healing and nurturing power. Realize how important these foods are to every cell in your body. Take your time. Enjoy!

Make meal time a special time every night. Eat in your formal dining room, with no television or other stimulus except each family member's company and conversation. Use this time to catch up on how everyone's day went. Tell funny stories. Laugh. Cast off the worries or stressors of the day. Lose yourself in the comfort of home and good food.

How does the food smell? Eating slower than you normally do, to chew your food until its liquid, do you taste the fresh herbs, seasonings and essences in the various dishes? Your taste buds are stimulated. Your hearts are filled with joy and song. Every night is a good night. You are enjoying life!

After dinner, consider a cup of tea such as mint with lavender. The mint is stimulating and a great digestive aid. A mint tea with a hint of fresh ginger that will also aid digestion is often my choice. The flavor is strong and soothing at the same time. The slice of lemon that I like to have floating atop the cup is beautiful and functional. It too aids digestion.

The lavender is very relaxing. We should always feel relaxed and calm when we eat. Also, lavender is good for helping to lull us to sleep. Embrace fresh herbs and their powers. Add them to your foods to the flavor.

There are supplements that potentially benefit those of us with vitiligo. These include an all B complex, to give us the extra B vitamins that are shown lacking in people with vitiligo. Emergen-C packets that you can mix with water for a refreshing drink are rich in minerals as well. The packets add much needed vitamin C along with other nutrients, to ensure balance. An essential fatty acid supplement is a potentially good one for vitiligo. Chia oil or hemp oil capsules are a good bet. A wild fish oil supplement makes it easy to change up Omega 3 supplements, which I recommend. Probiotics and prebiotics are recommended as a part of your daily regimen. Also, apple cider vinegar, a digestive enzyme supplement and papaya tablets may prove helpful. These enzyme supplements are best used before a heavy protein meal, which includes fibrous beans or meat.

Picrorhiza has been shown to help reduce the size of vitiligo patches. It is an Auyervedic herb that I've used for many years. Picrorhiza is a potentially powerful liver cleanser and it stimulates T and B cell activity, often used for hepatitis, AIDS, autoimmune and other degenerative diseases, research shows.

Fermented foods are good for your health. Apple cider vinegar is a staple in my diet, as is sauerkraut and other fermented foods. Fermented foods encourage a healthful gut flora. A spoonful of apple cider vinegar before eating a high protein meal is shown to aid digestion and absorption.

Fermented foods are shown to help to create beneficial bacteria in our gut, which keeps harmful bacteria and parasites at bay. It is important to include fermented foods in your daily diet. A simple salad dressing that includes apple cider vinegar, with mother of vinegar, is an easy way to add more fermented foods to your diet.

Living healthfully doesn't mean deprivation. There are many healthful desserts, from halving apples or pears, drizzled with agave sweetener mixed with cloves, cinnamon and nutmeg and baking for 30 minutes. Also, making your own ice cream is fun with electric ice cream freezers. Substituting coconut milk for cow's milk, and agave for sugar, create a potentially healthful, gut-loving treat. Making a sorbet of orange juice and frozen bananas blended is a nice ending to a meal. There are countless ways to incorporate healthful foods into the most tempting desserts, without the use of sugar or gluten.

A healthful dessert may include coconut kefir, a fermented dairy-like product that is highly beneficial to a well-balanced intestinal flora. I like Kefir with a hint of fresh vanilla bean and agave. Agave has prebiotics such as inulin and FOS, as well as a low-glycemic index. Served over sprouted granola, that includes raisins, raw pecans, and dates, and a sprinkling of freshly grated cinnamon bark. Garnishing with an edible mint leaf atop the dessert makes the dish as beautiful and appetizing as it is healthful.

Alkalinity is key to health! The food choices we make have a great impact on our acid to alkaline blood chemistry. As mentioned earlier, we can affect alkalinity through the skin with baths! Yes, bathing may help to balance acid-alkaline chemistry. Mixing a cup of Epsom salt with baking soda in a tub of water, then soaking for 30 minutes may help to remove acids from your body. This is a great way to de-stress before bed. This is a wonderful sleep aid to implement, as you relax in the warm tub of soothing and skin-softening alkalizing supplements. Epsom salts are rich in magnesium, which aids in relaxation. If your tub has jets, turn them on and enjoy the water massage! When you step out of your alkalizing bath, before you grab a towel, apply nutrients to your skin. Vitiligo Herbal Skin Cream, with a hint of fresh lavender, if it is bedtime, massaged into your body, from head to toe, helps to potentially heal, soothe and induce sleep. This is a great tool to implement. Remember, your skin is your largest organ. Pampering the skin is very conducive to relaxation, and relaxation is very good for digestion and vitiligo!

Instead of coffee, consider more healthful after dessert drinks like tea or herbal alternatives to coffee. Though coffee has some powerful health benefits, it can also cause health problems. Coffee is shown to impede digestion and to add extra acid to the system, upsetting the acid-alkaline balance that we must have for proper digestion and optimal health. Warm chicory with almond milk and a hint of vanilla, slightly sweetened with agave is a potentially healthier alternative. It is a marvelous coffee substitute that also has probiotics and is often used as a blood detoxifier. If you are not quite ready to give up coffee just yet, consider going half and half with chicory and coffee, increasing chicory as time goes on, until you no longer need coffee in your diet.

Some potentially helpful detoxifying agents include bentonite clay, charcoal capsules and artesian water, for these are detoxifying agents that will serve you well in your life changing detoxifying processes. Please schedule a consultation to choose a detoxification program that is best for you.

It is my sincere hope that you have learned lots of things that will improve your digestion, health and vitiligo. Rolaids, Tums and other digestive aids are not a choice for me. These products may further lower stomach acid, causing even more health problems. Live healthful foods, pure water, happy relationships, fulfilling jobs and a well-balanced life, all play a role in digestion, health and longevity.

Make a commitment to a healthful overall lifestyle, including eating right, exercising, spending time with people you like and love, doing what you are passionate about, in terms of work. Take the time to play, laugh, and live life to its fullest! These are the keys to good digestion and health. You own the key! Make the changes necessary to live!

To recap, I recommend drinking plenty of water, herbal teas and fruit juices, preferably fresh squeezed, for proper digestion. Vegetables, fruits, seeds, nuts and other foods in their raw state give us an infusion of vitamins, minerals, phytonutrients and enzymes that are essential to healthful digestion and disease prevention.

Daily supplements to ensure all nutritional needs are met is a way of life for me. Take the time to ensure you have a good vitamin and mineral supplement regimen. Probiotics, essential fatty acids, the herb picrorhiza and digestive enzymes are recommended as part of your daily regimen.

Ensuring proper stomach acid, with apple cider vinegar, lemon water, hydrochloric acid, if needed, and enzyme therapy will potentially help with food absorption.

Learn about the Broda Barnes basal temperature test for your thyroid, as well as the Heidelberg test for stomach acid deficiency. Find an endocrinologist you're comfortable with, as well as a nutritionally oriented medical doctor to monitor your overall health and nutrient levels.

I hope reading this book will give you a sense of empowerment! We are not defined by our spots or illnesses. We are defined by our determination to give our bodies what they need to return our skin color and health. That is our mission. That is our goal.

This book is written with passion, for educational purposes only.

I hope you find the information both inspiring and beneficial. Please give feedback on the

book on the VSIG blog
www.TheWellnessWell.net

Also, post comments to
facebook.com/vitiligoVSIG.

Your friendly naturopath and fellow vitiligo
sufferer,

Wanakee Hill, N.D.

Supplement Recommendations

Available @ www.TheWellnessWell.net

Wanakee's Naturopathics TM

Vitiligo Herbal Skin Cream.TM
Extra Strength

The most potent vitiligo herbal formula currently on the market, containing more active herbals that are shown to encourage re-pigmenting in the skin for faster results.

All Natural Herbal Cream
FDA's GMP (General Manufacturing Practices)
Quality control testing for purity and safety of all ingredients
No hidden ingredients
Safe and Effective for all skin types
90 Day Money Back Guarantee

Wanakee's Naturopathics TM

Vitiligo Herbal Skin Cream.™
Extra Strength

Ingredients: Coconut oil, Psoralea, Black Cumin Seed, Beeswax, Barberry, Calendula, PABA, Lavender

Coconut Oil is anti fungal and absorbing, allowing the herbal cream to penetrate the deeper inner layers of skin.

Psoralea increases the skin's photosensitivity, allowing the sun's UV rays to penetrate white vitiligo patches to encourage re-pigmenting.

Black Cumin Seed is a powerful and nutrient rich anti-inflammatory that is rich in Omega 3 fatty acids. Black Cumin Seed is used since ancient times to heal the skin and body.

Beeswax is an all natural skin protectant and sealant. Baby bees cannot produce honey. Their immature systems produce beeswax instead. This nutrient dense wax seals the honey into the beehive to prevent bacteria and contamination. The beeswax facilitates healing as well as sealing the herbal cream onto the vitiligo white patches to help ensure herbal absorption and more effective healing.

Barberry is an antibacterial herb used for centuries to facilitate healing in skin disorders.

Calendula is an herbal anti-inflammatory used to heal vitiligo and other skin diseases and trauma.

PABA is a natural B vitamin and sun screen that is shown to encourage re-pigmentation of white vitiligo patches.

Lavender adds a relaxing aroma that may enduce sleep and lower tension.

Available @ <u>www.TheWellnessWell.net</u>

Thymic Protein A sublingual protein powder for immune balance/hair growth/vitiligo support/accelerated healing

Ultra Raw Thyroid and **Iodoral**® for thyroid nourishment/metabolism/vitiligo and glandular support

Ultra Raw Adrenal Cortex for adrenal nourishment/stress/vitiligo support

Ultra Raw Pancreas for pancreas nourishment/metabolism of proteins and carbohydrates/vitiligo support

Homeopathic Ignatia Amara for stress relief and vitiligo

Homeopathic Bio Plasma for balancing body salts, vitiligo, anti-aging and overall health

Slimming Tea for detoxification support, weight loss, cleansing and purifying

Honey & Black Seed
Bar Soap - Body Wash - Lotion

Other *Supplement Recommendations*

Available at www.iherb.com

Use **discount code WAN856 for $5 off** first order.

Multiple Vitamin/Mineral Complex

B complex vitamin with a Sublingual B 12

Picrorhiza for vitiligo, digestion, liver detoxification, immune balancing, nutrient absorption, anti-aging and general health

Triphala

Vitamin D 3

Ginseng

B12 packets

Omega 3 fatty acids

Vitamin C Ascorbate

Ginkgo Biloba

Lavender and other essential oils

References & Recommended Reading

Agaston, A. (2003). *The south beach diet.* Emmaus, PA: Rodale Press

Balch, J.F. & Balch, P.A. (1997). *Prescription for nutritional healing.* Garden City Park, New York: Avery Publishing Group

Beardsley, T. Thymic Protein-A published in Journal of the National Academy of Sciences (Vol. 80, pp 6005-6009, October 1983, Immunology).

Campbell, T.C. & Campbell, T.M. (2006). *The china study.* Dallas, TX: Benbella Books

Carper, J. (2000). *Your miracle brain.* New York: HarperCollins Publishers

Diet to help eliminate anxiety retrieved from: from www.homeopathic.com/store/ntp/**stress**.jsp

Fermented foods: retrieved from http://www.healingcrow.com/ferfun/ferfun.html

Gladstar, R. (2008) *Rosemary Gladstar's herbal recipes for vibrant* health. North Adams, MA: Storey

Garrett, J.T. (2003). The Cherokee herbal. Rochester, Vermont: Bear and Company

Ginkgo Biloba article retrieved from: http://www.umm.edu/altmed/articles/ginkg o-biloba-000247.htm

Gittleman, A.L., (2002), The fat flush plan. New York: McGraw Hill

Haas, E. & Levin, B. (2006) *Staying healthy with nutrition.* Berkley, CA: Celestial Arts

Hobday, R. (2004). *The healing sun.* Scotlan, UK: Findhorn Press

Hyman, M. (2006). Ultra – Metabolism. New York: Scribner

Kushi, M. (1995). *Guide to standard macrobiotic diet.* Becket, MA: One Peaceful World Press

Lindlahr, H. (1919). *Philosophy of natural therapeutics.* Chicago: The Lindlahr Publishing Co.

Lipski, E. (2005) *Digestive Wellness. New York,* NY: McGraw-Hill

Mitchell, S. (2001). *A practical guide to naturopathy.* Columbus, Ohio: Custom Publishing.

Montes, L. ((2006) *Vitiligo current knowledge & nutritional therapy.* Buenos Aires, Argentina: Westhoven Press

Omega 3 Fatty Acid article retrieved from
http://www.jacn.org/cgi/content/abstract/2
1/6/495

Page, L. (2006) *Linda Page's healthy healing*.
Carmel Valley, CA: Healthy Healing Inc.

PABA & Vitiligo retrieved from VSIG archives:
http://listserv.icors.org/scripts/wa-icors.exe

Pfeiffer, C.C. (1987). *Nutrition and mental illness*.
Rochester, VT: Healing Arts Press

Salaman, M. *Foods that heal. Maximum
Publishing*

Stoll, A.L. (2001). *The omega 3 connection*. New
York: Simon and Schuster

Stress and Anxiety retrieved from:
http://www.ecomii.com/pregnancy-
problems/insomnia

Summerfield, L.M. (2001. *Nutrition, exercise and
behavior*. Belmont, CA: Wadsworth Thomson
Learning

Tierra, M. (1998) *The way of herbs*. New York,
NY: Pocket Books

Williams, J.E. (2003) *Prolonging Health*.
Charlottesville, VA: Hampton Roads
Publishing Company, Inc.

www.avrf.org/facts/sun.htm

Retrieved from Variant of *TYR* and
Autoimmunity Susceptibility Loci in
Generalized Vitiligo
Y. Jin and Others

Retrieved from http://www.vegetarian-
nutrition.info/phprint.php

Retrieved from
http://www.sciencedirect.com/science?_ob=
ArticleURL&_udi=B6WBF-4C6JK2J-
6&_user=10&_coverDate=04%2F30%2F2004&_
rdoc=1&_fmt=high&_orig=search&_sort=d&_
docanchor=&view=c&_searchStrId=133003077
1&_rerunOrigin=google&_acct=C000050221&_
version=1&_urlVersion=0&_userid=10&md5=
575aced02d20ad19a52f317b60e91810

Retrieved from
thyroid.about.com/od/gettestedanddiagnosed
/a/bloodtests.htm

Retrieved from
http://www.ncbi.nlm.nih.gov/pmc/articles/
PMC1431557/table/T1/

Rodale Press Books that my mom ordered via
mail in my teen years

Made in the USA
Charleston, SC
20 January 2011